THE COMPLETE GUIDE TO AIRPORT EXERCISE

by

KEN SEIFERT

TP

TELEMACHUS PRESS

THE COMPLETE GUIDE TO AIRPORT EXERCISE

Cover designed by Telemachus Press, LLC

Cover art:
Copyright © iStockPhoto/174931314/chinaface
Copyright © iStockPhoto/187025827_PeopleImages
Copyright © iStockPhoto/539649154/panic_attack
Copyright © iStock_176200506_1MoreCreative

Interior photographs Copyright © Ken Seifert

Published by Telemachus Press, LLC
http://www.telemachuspress.com

Visit the author website:
http://www.facebook.com/airportexercise

ISBN: 978-1-945330-60-5 (eBook)
ISBN: 978-1-945330-61-2 (Paperback)

HEALTH & FITNESS

10 9 8 7 6 5 4 3 2 1

Version 2017.08.11

For Jeremy, who would never have exercised in airports
if he hadn't met me.

Note from Author:

I am literally in an airport as I write the first few sentences of this book. Having just completed 30 sets of squats and 50 sets of shoulder exercises in addition to some stomach crunches, the idea of airport exercise is as routine for me as getting delayed on my American Airlines flight from Miami to Santo Domingo.

What makes me qualified to provide advice on working out in airports? I have been successfully doing it in more than 50 domestic and international airports for the last 15 years. And while there are numerous websites, blogs, and articles that provide *some* fitness tips for exercising in airports, this is the first comprehensive "manual" that provides step by step instructions on how to make a workout effective and successful. From getting the right, low maintenance equipment to cleaning up afterwards so you aren't "that guy" with killer body odor whose seatmates wish you would get lost, this book will give you the tips and guidance on how to get moving during your layovers.

As a U.S. Foreign Service Officer (fancy word for diplomat), traveling through airports around the country and world is like second nature. I can tell you where to find the best Cuban sandwich in any airport (La Carreta in the Miami International Airport) and where to find the best USO military lounges (Denver International Airport and Chicago O'Hare come to mind). And, I have perfected my workout regime, studying how to most effectively exercise in airports during layovers, both short and long.

Okay, truth be told, I guess you could say I am an exercise fiend. I work out 2.5-3 hours a day minimum, every day, always. No exceptions. I even found ways to exercise on a small 16 passenger dual-hulled boat which spent 6 days at sea, traveling around the Galapagos Islands. And while most of the world isn't this obsessed (most of the world also doesn't also eat an entire batch of brownies in one sitting either), exercise is a critical ingredient to one's overall health.

Also, I really hate wasting time, which is why I only commute to work by bicycle, almost never by car since the traffic where I live is quite intense. Anyone who has flown over the Christmas holiday or during a winter storm at the Omaha airport (and gotten stuck) knows that flight delays and long layovers result in many wasted hours. Think of how many days of your life you will have spent in airports, waiting for your flight to take off. Couldn't those hours have been better spent?

Over the years, my airport exercising has sparked much conversation among my friends and family, but also with countless, random people who watch me as I run past them in the terminals with my headphones or feverishly try to fit in a few extra resistance cords sets before my boarding begins. Ahh, I probably don't have to rush since I am in Group 5 boarding—thanks, Delta Airlines!

I promised myself that when the 100th person made a comment, asked a question, or said something about my airport workouts, I would write this book. Well, that benchmark finally came as I was about to board a red-eye flight from Denver to Miami on my way back to the Dominican Republic. A rather portly man under a wool blanket, sleeping on the floor of Gate A49, looked up and said, "Wow son—you gotta keep it up. You should write a book and get us to exercise." He then farted and went back to sleep.

So, writing it all down I shall do. Bearing in mind that I am not a medical doctor and am not a professional fitness trainer, this book is not meant to be a step by step guide on correct exercise form or what your resting heart rate should be. Talk to professionals about these things, like your doctor, before you start exercising. This book is about practical steps and tips on how to exercise in airports and transform your lifestyle that will likely grow beyond just these layover workouts.

Lastly, I would say that like anything else in life, using common sense is the name of the game. Following rules, listening to those in charge, respecting your surroundings, and having a keen situational awareness are "musts" as you endeavor to bring exercise routines into busy and crowed airports. But like that famous saying goes, the world makes way for men and women who know where they are going, and they are often rewarded with fresh, delicious donuts. I am paraphrasing of course.

Table of Contents

THE COMPLETE GUIDE TO AIRPORT EXERCISE

CHAPTER I
Why Bother?

WHETHER YOU'RE STUCK for 30 minutes waiting for your plane or you have a 5-hour layover in some airport, there are many healthy choices for passing the time. But most people just don't think about it or figure it's too hard or too much work to do anything meaningful during this commuting.

Flying takes time away from things you'd ordinarily want (or need) to do, like exercise. And while you may plan to do your workout when you get to your destination, how often do you arrive tired, with a list of "chores" you have to do, like running to the store, getting some food, or getting ready for that conference or board meeting? Working out is often first on the chopping block when more important things like family, eating, and appointments take over as higher priorities.

But the benefits of exercise are indisputable, for your heart, your mental state, and your overall fitness. So why not use that otherwise wasted time in airports to do something productive and healthy? Not only does this burn calories and get the blood flowing, which is important for overall health and fitness, but there is compelling evidence that having more limber muscles and joints is healthier when you finally board that airplane (reducing the risk for clots, restless leg syndrome, and soreness).

Anyone with a Netflix addition (like me) or a Smartphone knows it's easy to talk yourself out of exercise when there are more entertaining or tempting options. This is especially true in airports given how many other distractions there are and how overwhelming everything can be. The airport is filled with tired, grumpy, and often smelly people, so finding that quiet, empty corner to block it all out and listen to music or catch up on that book sounds really good. And sometimes that is just what the doctor ordered.

But when you really weigh how to best maximize the time spent idly in airports, consider all your options. Obviously, you could sit and do nothing, which may be refreshing at times (and maybe you just need the rest), but it can also be a complete waste of time. You can sit and judge people, wishing that loud family with the infant baby would quiet down or the group of ladies with their 14 bags would find some other place to sit. You could shop and spend an exorbitant amount of money on things you don't need like cigars or specialty chocolates or a new super charged set of headphones. You can eat and do some more eating—caving into those super-sized fries or authentic empanadas. Go ahead—indulge, but how long before your waistline hops a zip code?

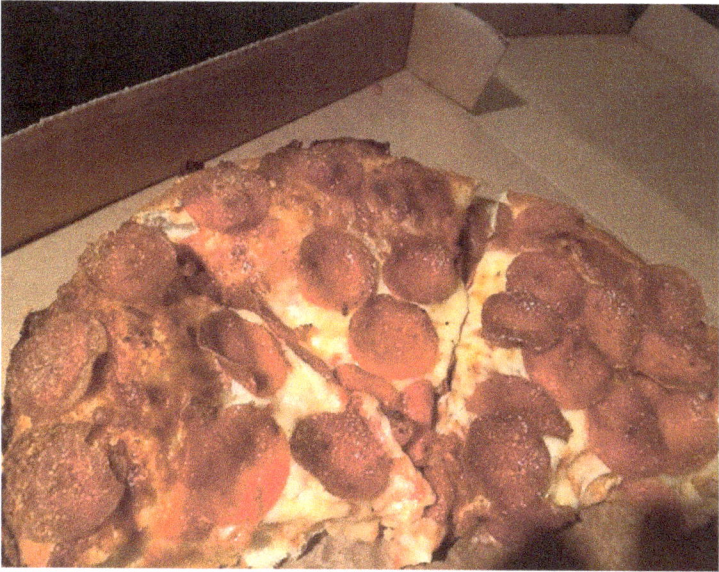

Or, you can consider the better option: get off your butt and go sweat. Your doctor will thank you, your loved ones (who remember how fit and young you used to be) will thank you, and most importantly, you will thank you. Think of the time you will save NOT having to hit the gym upon arriving at your spring break destination (okay maybe it's just exercise-crazed people like me that would even think that, but you get the idea). With this book, the time you spend in airports exercising will become routine and easy, and the benefits are plentiful.

CHAPTER II
Getting Started

AS MANY EXERCISE experts will tell you, think about what it is you want to accomplish. Do you just want to burn some calories? Do you want to stay on track with your established exercise routine; if it's "chest and triceps" day, for example, wouldn't you rather NOT mess up your routine for the week due to travel? Do you want to work up a really good sweat—not a mere glistening, but the kind that would make your high school gym coach proud? Or do you simply want to work off a bite or two of that Dunkin' Donut you bought? Hey it was right next to your terminal ... well ... okay who's kidding who, you ventured 28 gates out of your way just to get that perfectly glazed goodness, and I don't blame you!

It's helpful to have these goals in mind so you can better analyze your options and shape the kind of airport exercise that fits your lifestyle and priorities.

Do Some Research

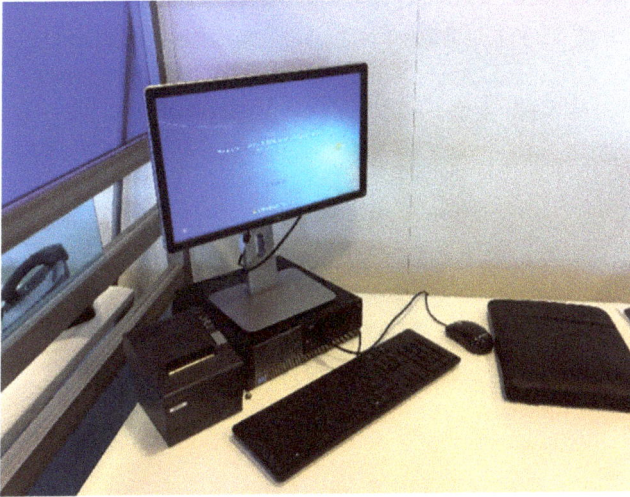

Once you have an idea of what your goals are, consider your options. In other words, do some research! Google the airport you will be flying through, and get the lay of the land. What's in the airport, and how are the terminals situated? Is the local city nearby? What kinds of gyms exist at or near the airport? Are you traveling to a small airport with limited real estate—as in running space? I recall flying in and out of the South Bend, Indiana airport for years; let's just say in terms of size, that airport is in no rush to becoming the next Atlanta Hartsfield-Jackson.

Having an idea of what the airport and local area can offer doesn't require creating complicated databases or even writing anything down. If you have time to read that news article on Jennifer Aniston's "real" thoughts on Angelina Jolie, then you can spare some time to educate yourself on the airport through which you are transiting.

And of course, always be mindful of your time. Knowing how long the security lines get in the airport, when the boarding starts (it does vary by airline), any extra steps required (if you are flying internationally for example), and of course how long you will take to clean up your sweaty self are all questions to ponder so you can adequately plan your workout.

Exercise Boosts Brainpower
Not only does exercise improve your body, it helps your mental function, says certified trainer David Atkinson.

Web MD

Packing

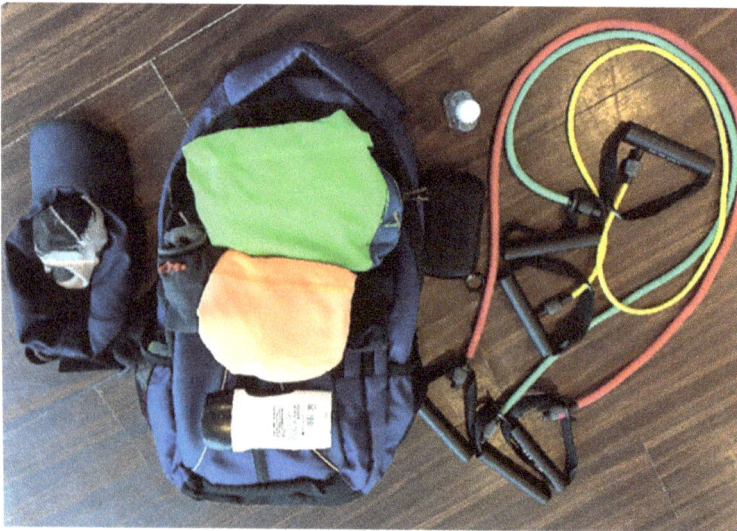

I hate to check any bags. The thought of being delayed upon arriving at my destination by having to wait for a bag makes me thoroughly annoyed. I recall some friends that we traveled with to the beautiful Seychelles Islands were delayed more than an hour at baggage claim. Being the good friends we are, we took the first bus departing the airport to our hotel and kindly left our friends to sort out their business and meet us there.

There are lots of tips for packing more sensibly. This is why, for example, I've invested in quick-wash underwear (REI has some good brands) that I can clean and reuse quickly, in that order. This underwear can be easily washed in a hotel sink, and they dry remarkably fast. Since you only need two pairs (one to wear, one to dry), this cuts down on bag space. I also try to be a minimalist with my travel items, including wearing my running shoes on the plane (vs. packing them) and not bringing more clothes than necessary as I can wear the same tie on two different days during a week-long business trip, for example (no one will know!).

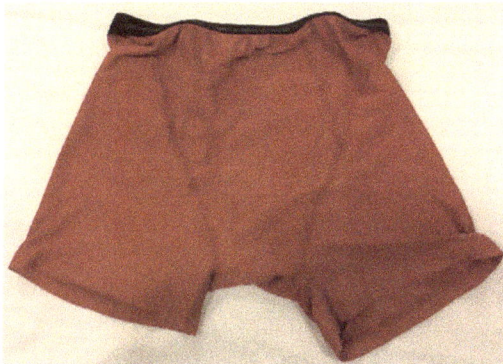

Whatever your taste or needs, you can often find ways to pack lighter, which allows you more flexibility and freedom to do your airport workouts. So, if family or travel buddies can't watch your bag, no problem. Running with a small backpack just means you are increasing the difficulty of your airport run by adding on some extra weight, which can be a good thing so long as you don't get your backpack too sweaty!

Packing travel size toiletries is a great way to save space and reduce weight. Everything from toothpaste to deodorant comes in a convenient travel size. In the Hygiene section, I'll offer more specific ideas on must-bring toiletries. Now, I know a lot of my female friends have said to me over the years that their toiletry needs are different, and that packing lightly is just not that easy. And yes, depending on the person and where she is flying to or what she plans on doing at her final destination, packing really lightly might not always be possible. But as I will explain later, you can easily and safely leave your items in the airport baggage storage office, which most large airports have.

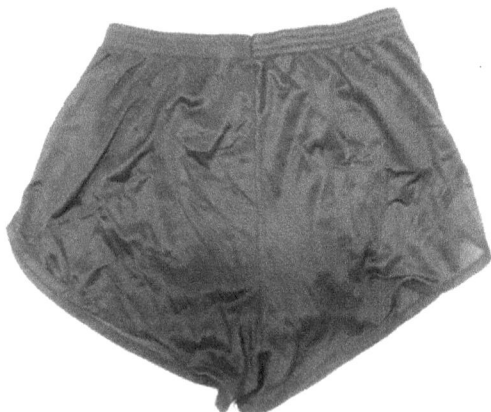

Another tip: wear your workout clothes under your regular clothes when you get to the airport; this also saves space and time. I have found that it makes sense to wear a pair of running shorts under my pants when I travel—the kind with inner lining so the shorts essentially serve as your underwear too (particularly useful for men). This saves space as well as time when you get to the airport, as you don't need a bathroom to change but can simply remove your pants. There are all kinds of brands of running shorts, from the long baggy styles to the less modest Soffe versions that actually are quite light weight, comfortable, and don't bunch. Just be prepared to get a few looks if you wear those bad boys while working out in the airport; they often leave little to the imagination.

Less than 5% of adults participate in 30 minutes of physical activity each day, and only one in three adults receives the recommended amount of physical activity each week.

https://www.fitness.gov

CHAPTER III
Airport Gyms

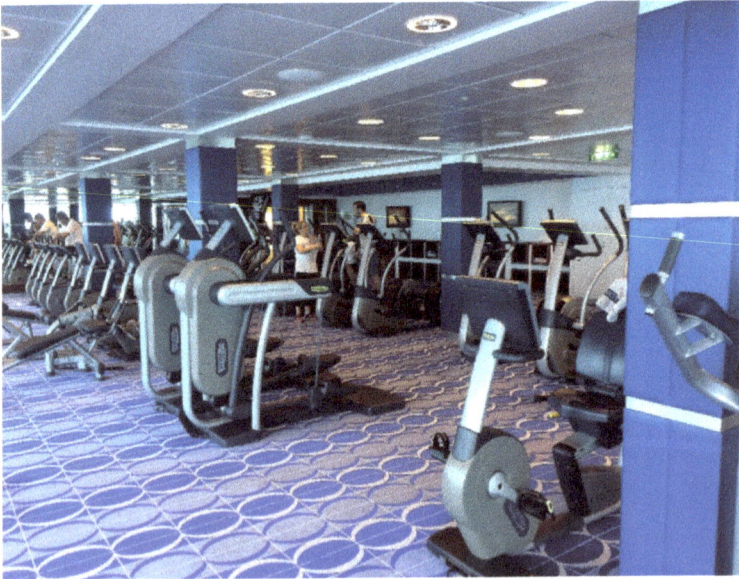

BEAR IN MIND that many airports actually house gyms or fitness centers or even yoga studios that make exercising relatively easy. In many airports, like Baltimore-Washington International, you can easily find gyms located in nearby hotels or those in the local vicinity. By doing a quick google search, you can often find a gym located just a few miles from the airport. There are several websites that can point you in the right direction, including: http://www.airportgyms.com and even some apps for your Smartphone which give you all the information you might need about gym options.

With dozens of airport gyms in the United States alone, and even more at international airports, this may be your best bet. The pros: many of these gyms have a diversity of equipment, showers, and the privacy of working out without getting odd stares from your fellow airport-goers. The cons really come down to the three Cs: the cost, the crowds, and the extra time for commuting (if you opt to leave the airport for a nearby gym). Just as I do in life, let me focus on the negatives first so you know what to expect.

Gym Costs

While the G-Force Health Club in Dubai may only cost you $15 for admission for one hour, for example, other gyms like the Radisson Blu Hotel near the Zurich airport can set you back nearly $25 or more (at least the last time I checked). While there is usually a fee in an airport or nearby gym, many facilities (especially Bally's, LA Fitness, YMCA, and Gold's Gym) may offer 1 or 2 week "trials" that allow you free access for a limited period. Usually you just print a trial membership form from the gym's website. But be prepared for the gym attendants to try to "sell" you on the gym when you arrive, hoping you will buy an annual membership. That can be a major time killer, and you might have to politely say you are not interested. Remember that these free trials can't usually be repeated at the same location.

Gym Crowds

There's no guarantee the gym in the airport will be empty enough to really get in a good workout. If you have dozens of sweaty, fellow passengers trying to get in a few sets on the seated butterfly machine or if that woman from Cincinnati has been hogging the 15-pound dumbbells for 20 minutes, you may find the gym experience is too crowded and frustrating to really meet your exercise goals.

Gym Commuting

Also keep in mind that many of the gyms are not always in the actual airport; many are in hotels connected to the airport or near the airport, which means you may have to commute. For example, there is a Gold's Gym about three miles from the Miami Airport. Now, you could run to the gym from the airport saving money and getting your cardio in (more on that later), but even this takes time, and not everyone will be at the fitness level to do that. At Ronald Reagan National Airport in Washington DC, gyms are just a couple of metro stops away, including Pentagon City and Crystal City. But either way, this is extra time you will need to factor into everything.

Lastly, in terms of gym options, also bear in mind that for yoga lovers, novice or expert, many airports have different fitness options. The Dallas Fort Worth Airport (excellent for running) and San Francisco International Airport offer free yoga rooms, for example. Just don't pull your groin muscle doing that downward facing dog pose!

Less time sitting is associated with better sleep and health. Those who sit for fewer than 8 hours a day were significantly more likely to report "very good" sleep quality. Exercising at any time of the day appears to be good for sleep. Contrary to long-standing "sleep hygiene" advice, exercising close to bedtime was not associated with poorer sleep quality. In fact, exercise was linked to better sleep no matter what time of day.

https://sleepfoundation.org

The bottom line, there are pros to using airport gyms (and gyms near the airport). This is a rather convenient way to squeeze a workout in, but as I mentioned, you have to consider the variables. Do you have time to leave the airport to get to the gym? Sure, you can probably manage to take a taxi from La Guardia Airport in New York City to any number of gyms nearby, but do you have the time to return to the airport and go back through security? Are you willing to consider the costs of the gym itself and possibly a taxi ride if you can't safely run to and from that airport?

Just get online and see what you find. For those who have some money to burn and are looking for a quick, no-nonsense way to exercise during your layover, gyms are an excellent option.

CHAPTER IV
Airport Workouts for Dummies

FOR EVERYONE ELSE, I'm here to provide some realistic tips for how to successfully complete a workout in the airport. Many blogs and opinion pieces out there will talk about sequestering yourself in small corner of the airport and stretching. Stretching can be a great thing indeed. So can walking around the terminals or using your bag to do some light weight-lifting. Think of the bag as a big weight you can use to work those arms, shoulders, and back.. If you are in the market for more of strenuous workout, help is here.

Resistance Cords

One of the best pieces of exercise equipment I ever purchased is standard resistance cords (bands). This is truly the most under-appreciated exercise equipment on the planet. These cords, a relatively small item, usually fit neatly in a tiny bag smaller than most purses. They can give you a vast array of workout options which you can do almost anywhere. This may include standing in line at the grocery store, which I have done, or killing some time as you acclimate on your hike up Mt. Kilimanjaro; yep, I brought the cords with me then too!

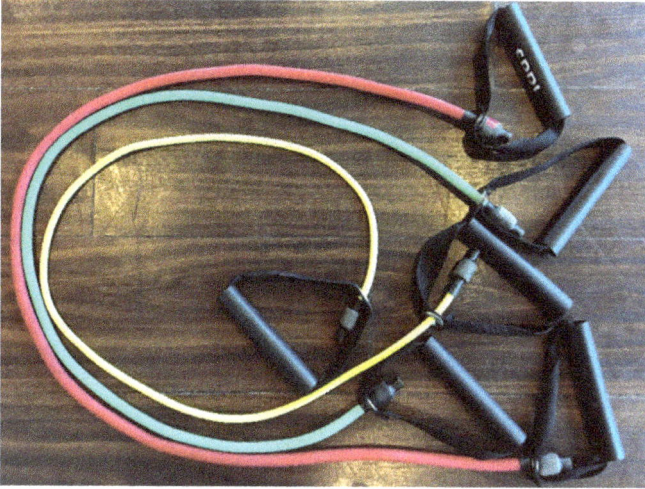

These cords can be used to exercise all your core muscle groups and can even substitute for a gym during periods in your life where you simply don't have access to one. As a relatively poor college student studying abroad in Santiago, Chile for six months, this exercise lifeline provided the framework of my upper body workouts. I may not have been ripped like the Rock, but I was more than sufficiently fit.

Perhaps most impressive is the fact you can take these cords in your suitcase to use almost anywhere including hotels, airports, and even airplanes themselves. As far as airplanes, this really ends up depending on the flight attendants. On long international flights, in particular, few flight attendants have bothered me about discreetly using my cords near a bathroom or near my seat. The same goes for doing 90-degree leg squats. As long as I am not blocking the aisle or standing up when the "fasten seatbelt" light is on, airline crew rarely hassle me when I use my cords. In fact, many have expressed real interest and fascination in my mini work outs. Some even vowed to start doing the same. But when in doubt, ask, and always follow the direction of those in charge.

While there are many brands to choose from (a simple Amazon.com search will give you the options), I have found Gofit Pro Gym to be the most durable—which run about $25. They come with multiple bands which allow you to customize your amount of resistance. Sets often contain 20, 30, and 40-pound bands that you can add on to increase the resistance. If you don't have enough resistance, it isn't really a great workout, so add/remove bands until you get the right amount.

Exercise puts the spark back into your sex life

Regular physical activity can improve energy levels and physical appearance, which may boost your sex life. Regular physical activity may enhance arousal for women. And men who exercise regularly are less likely to have problems with erectile dysfunction than are men who don't exercise.

http://www.mayoclinic.org

While there are dozens of different cords, in multiple colors with varied grips, my advice is to not go too cheap as repeated use may eventually break the bands; so you might as well go for the higher quality.. Hey, if the cords do end up breaking eventually, after repeated and long term use, this just means you are using the cords in a meaningful way.

While online websites give you the full range of exercise options with resistance cords, let's go over a few basics:

By standing about two feet apart (depending on your height), with both of your feet planted right on the middle of the cords and with one hand on each handle grip, you can curl upwards in controlled motions to work your biceps. Remember to curl well beyond 90 degree angles towards your body to get the full range of muscle use.

Diagram 1: Bicep curl

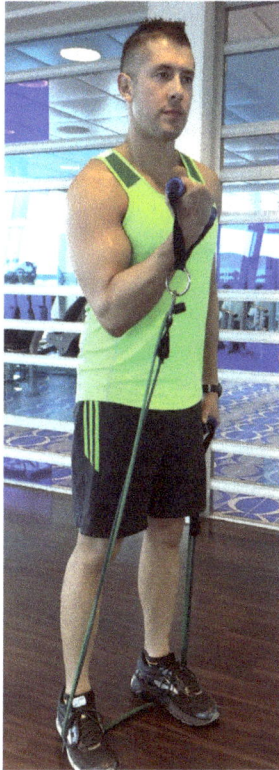

Or putting your feet in the same position, you can adjust the direction of your curl, pulling the cords diagonally towards your chest, crossing the cords first with your right hand curling the cords towards your left pectoral (pec) and left hand curling the cords towards your right pec. Or you can curl both hands at the same time. These exercises can work those pec muscles as well as biceps.

Diagram 2: Pectoral crossover curls

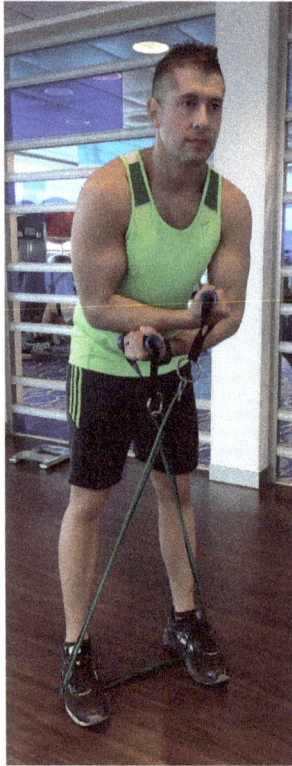

Lifting the cords handles upwards in a steady, controlled motion towards your chin gives those shoulders a workout. You should try to lift the cords beyond a 90-degree angle with your shoulders. It may not be as good as the free weights, but resistance exercise can produce surprising results.

Diagram 3: Shoulder raises

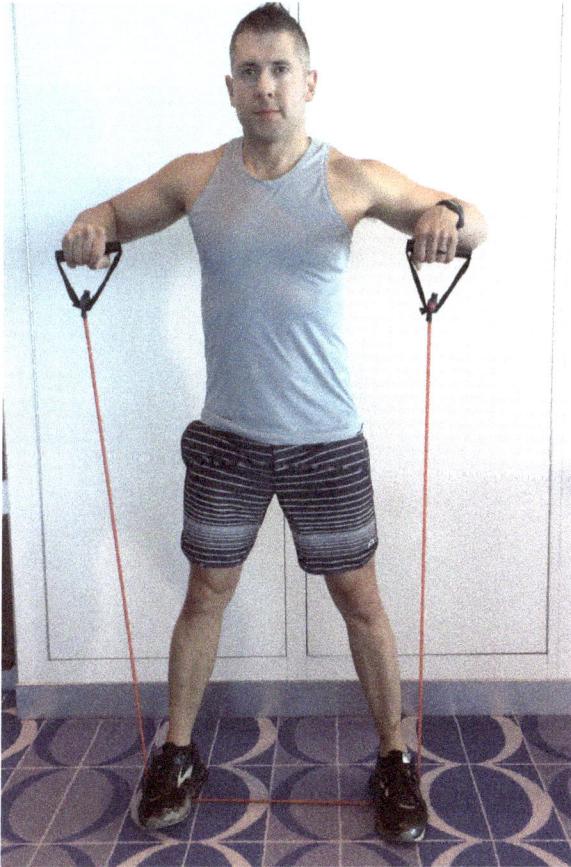

Another option: grab the cord handles in each hand, wrapping the cords around your hand once each, and pull outwards like your opening up curtains, starting directly in front of your face and then back again (you guessed it, this works those back muscles).

Diagram 4: Lateral (back) extensions

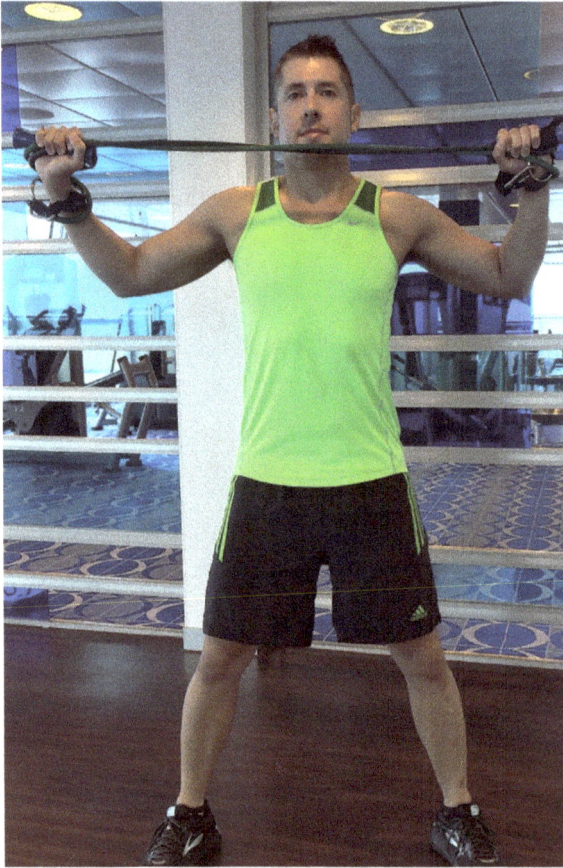

You can start with 5 or 10 sets per muscle group with about 8-10 repetitions or reps. This can easily turn into a 20-minute workout to get the blood flowing and tear some of those muscle fibers, in a good way! Or you can go a bit harder and longer (especially during those 4-5 hour layovers in Newark) and do 50-60 sets per muscle group. This can become an hour or more of working out. You can use the resistance cords to work all of your major muscle groups. Usually the resistance cords come with additional diagrams and recommendations for exercises, and you can find more information online.

Squats

In addition, you need not neglect the legs! You can do basic squats anywhere. That is, from a standing position, bend your knees to a 90-degree angle, making sure to stick your backside out as you "squat" down and come back up. Be careful that your knees don't go beyond the edge of your toes. You can either put your hands behind your head as you squat down or you can grab one of your carry-on bags and hold that over your head or out in front of you as you do the squats. This will work your legs harder and burn even more calories! You can do 10 sets of 10 or 30 sets of 10, and this will give you a decent leg workout. And as mentioned above, you'd be surprised how little space this takes—including on an airplane. Just remember to move in a controlled and steady way, as your knees and back should be treated with respect and consideration. You might even go on YouTube and study proper form before trying.

The mental benefits of aerobic exercise have a neurochemical basis. Exercise reduces levels of the body's stress hormones. It also stimulates the production of endorphins, chemicals in the brain that are the body's natural painkillers and mood elevators. Endorphins are responsible for the "runner's high" and for the feelings of relaxation and optimism that accompany many hard workouts.

http://www.health.harvard.edu

Diagram 5: Simple Leg Squats

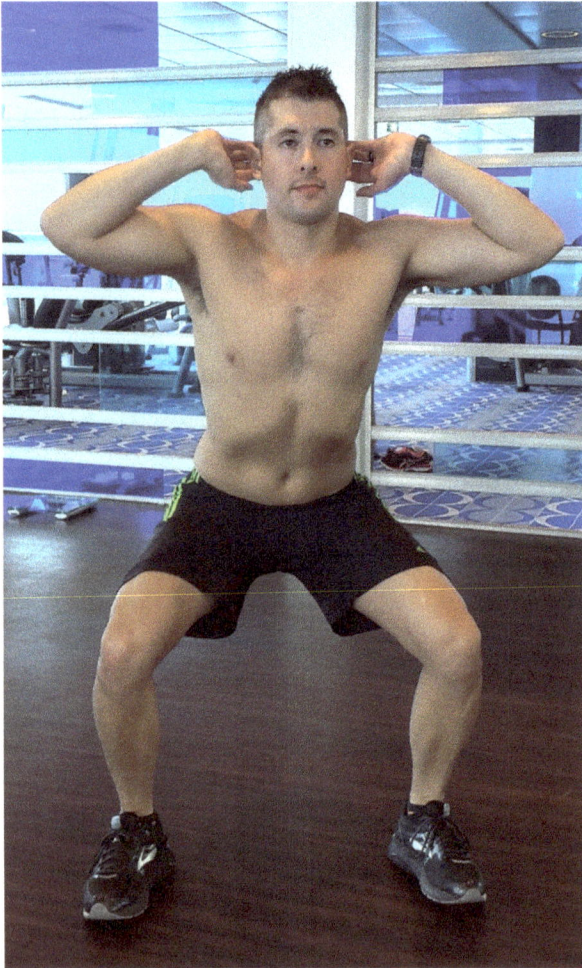

And if you want to work those calves some more, you can stand straight with your feet shoulder-length apart, and raise yourself up and down using your calf muscles in sets of 10 or 20. This is actually something you can do almost anywhere; I do calf-raises when I am brushing my teeth, standing in line, and on planes. I don't recommend doing it when you are trying to pee, however. It doesn't end well.

Using the Airport Chairs

These little suckers can do more than rest your aching butt. You can incorporate the chair as part of your workout, from triceps dips to stomach crunches. The internet can provide you with many different ideas and options. AnytimeFitness has a blog that talks about calf, hip, and glute stretches. Here are some common exercises one can do with the chairs.

Diagram 6: Tricep extensions

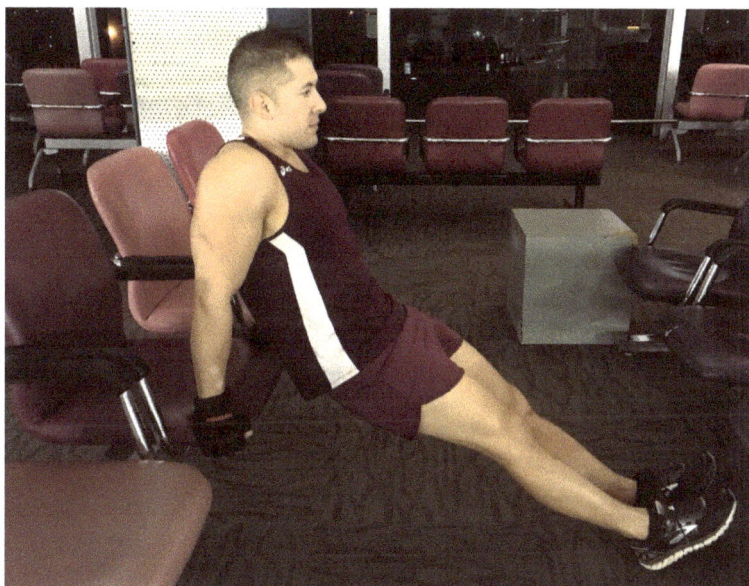

Perhaps the most popular exercise using airport chairs is the seated triceps dips. You start by placing your arms straight with your palms flat against the edge of your seat. Meanwhile, you extend your legs straight in front of you to allow your body to get a good range of motion as you dip downwards and upwards, working your triceps. The triceps are the biggest muscles in your arms and look significantly more toned when regularly exercised.

You can also combine some cardio exercises with muscle strengthening. For example, you can sit in the chair and raise your knees up towards your chest in a steady, controlled motion, one at a time working your stomach and quadriceps. Be mindful to keep your back straight and use your arms to steady your upper body so you don't put undue strain on your lower back. If you do this for ten minutes, and you will definitely get the blood flowing and sweat as well! You can also try to do all-out crunches if the seats don't have armrests. The angle may be a little awkward though, so be careful not to overstrain your lower back.

Want to work those pectoral muscles? You can do chair pushups easily and effectively. Simply place both palms facing downwards on the chairs, shoulder length apart. Meanwhile, extend your legs outward behind you, aligned with your back; remember to keep your back straight. Essentially, your body is in push-up form; only in this case, you are pushing off the chairs instead of the ground. Raise your body downward and then back up in slow, controlled motions, working those chest muscles.

Diagram 7: Raised push-ups

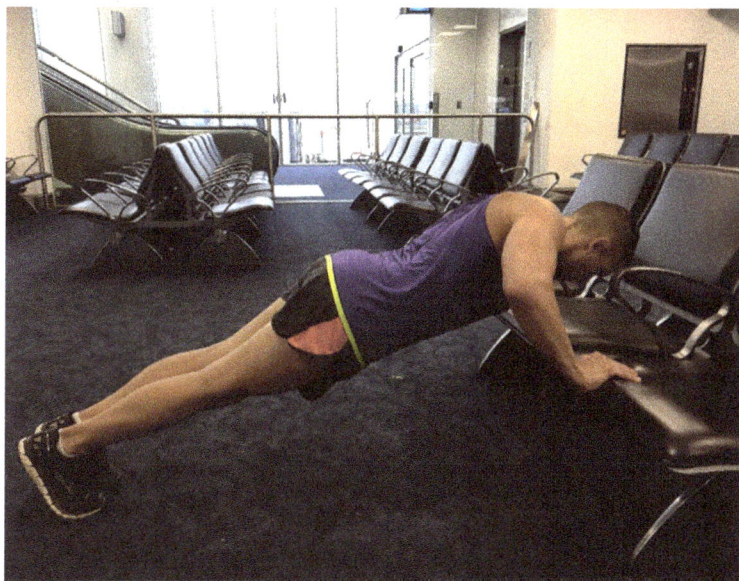

Other Airport Workouts

There are many exercises that you can do in the airport that involve resistance cords, the seat, and gravity. You can also consider going back to some of the basics, like jumping jacks. While this may bring you a little more attention than you might prefer, doing even ten minutes of jumping jacks or boxing (punching) exercises can burn those calories and get your heart racing. Just remember to stretch before you start exercising.

If you are able to find some relatively quiet (and maybe clean) part of the airport, you can even get more sophisticated and do some burpees. These are excellent exercise options that increase your core strength, flexibility, burn calories, and build muscles particularly in your quadriceps, back, and arms. I would recommend keeping a small towel (which you can bring with you in your bag) or some paper towels to wipe up your sweat and keep your workout area clean and hygienic for other passengers. To see more information about how a burpee works, check out YouTube.

Depending on where you travel, you might also find many diverse options for working out. Whether it's ice skating at the Seoul Incheon Airport or golfing near the Abu Dhabi airport or "art-walks" at the Seattle-Takoma International airport, you might find all kinds of activities that get the heart beating, and if you're lucky, give you a good, sustained workout.

With a little creativity, research, and planning, you can turn those wasted minutes at the airport into valuable exercise time that helps you relax and fly better once you actually get on the plane. And you might even deserve that reward later when you wake up bright and early in Rome.

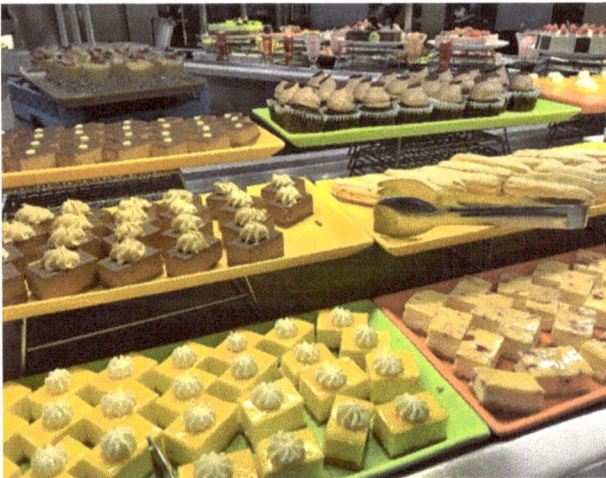

CHAPTER V
Running

RUNNING IN AND around airports is perhaps my favorite form of exercise during those long layovers. Those spacious, vast terminals offer more than just empty halls for bored tourists. They provide a very suitable running path, whether for a short jog or marathon training. You heard it—flying is no excuse to neglect your long runs! The Miami International Airport for example gives you ample space to complete that quick 5K. Just two laps from one end of the terminal to the other provides vast real estate to burn those calories (experts estimate you burn between 70-100 calories every 7 minutes of moderate running); this will help you keep your training up and exercise program on track.

From Dubai to Panama City, big airports or small, your run may not be the most exciting you will ever do, though running past Buddhists monks, Arab women in hijabs, a couple fighting with each other, and an international soccer team in the same 10-minute span, as happened to me in the Cairo airport once, can make airport-runs a truly memorable and cultural experience.

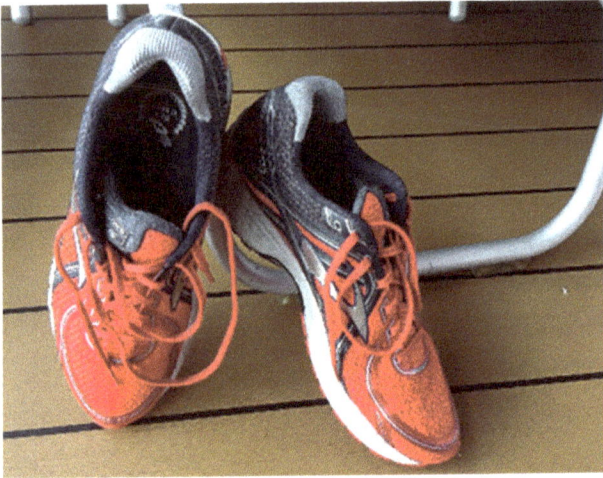

When people ask me about my running in airports, one of their first questions is, are you sure running is allowed? To answer this, I ask a couple of questions back. First, have you have ever been late for a flight? Or were you ever on a long layover, and those nachos left you feeling a bit unsettled, causing you to rush to the nearest toilet? What did you do in those situations? You RAN. Running happens all the time in airports, at all times of the day, and at all times of the year. Whether it's that mother racing after her 3-year-old son who just "has" to chase his ball down the terminal or those grandparents from Salt Lake City who fell asleep and missed the loud message over the airport intercom informing them their gate had changed, and it is now final boarding, people run in airports all the time.

Since running in airports is actually quite typical, why should you be any different? From Germany to the United States to El Salvador to Australia to Ethiopia to Uzbekistan, I have run in airports. As long as I am not over the top about it (that is, bumping into travelers who probably deserve it or knocking down flight attendants, who don't deserve it), no one really cares if you run.

In fact, as I run past airport security and TSA officials, with my sweaty shirt and headphones, I will often get a thumbs-up and smiles. All the same, do keep in mind the local culture of the place in which you run and the unique airport into which you fly. Ben Gurion airport in Tel Aviv, for example, may not be the best place to run because of the heightened security, but I have never tried running there!

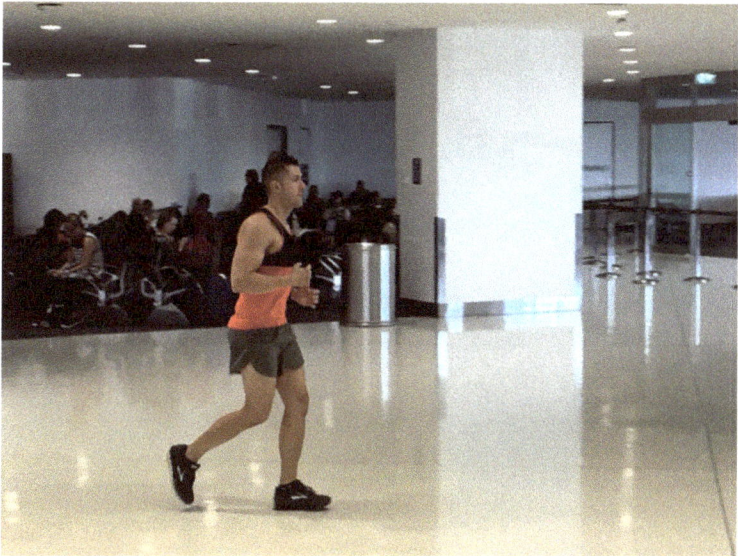

As you run from one end of the airport to the other, keep in mind that various hallways can take you into whole new areas of the airport. In the Panama City airport, for example, you can run towards various gates, then back towards the security screening area, then back towards another long hallway of gates, and by the end, you get in some serious mileage. In the Miami airport, you can use the stairs that lead up to the Skytrain as extra leg workouts. Go up and down one of those stair cases for 20 minutes, and you will break a sweat in no time; more, you will probably be alone on the stairs as most people opt for the adjacent escalator. Perhaps Frankfurt is the best example for great running space as the terminal halls are wide and clean and seem to go on forever.

Having run in airports for more than 15 years, I can honestly say I have never been stopped by anyone who had a problem with it. Though admittedly, I have "run" into people I knew, unexpectedly. I remember once, my former boss transiting from Angola to DC saw me running in the airport, waived, and called me over, which got a little awkward when I stopped and dripped sweat all over his shoes. I also "ran" into a former high school friend at LAX that I hadn't seen in almost 20 years; she was impressed to see me in such a fitness mode and said I looked great (so did she!).

Moderate *activity* *gets your heart beating faster, causes you to break a sweat and breathe harder—you should be able to talk but not sing.*

https://health.clevelandclinic.org

But in general, the stem of people naturally bends around you as you pass by. Just use caution, pay close attention to everything that's happening around you, especially those toads of people who stop all of a sudden in the middle of the hallway to look up their gate number, not caring who they block in the process. Don't they realize they are looking at the arrival screen, not the departures? Sure, sometimes airports can get a little crowded, and running comfortably is not an option. But even during crowded hours, there are still routes and parts of the terminal where you can find running room. You can wear headphones if that helps pump you up for the run, so long as it doesn't become distracting for you.

Running Near Airports

This is a great past-time and very doable. Again, just doing basic research can help you identify nearby running routes that open up a world of opportunity during those long lay-overs. Google Maps can point you in the right direction.

Often times, I find it fun to pick a destination in mind when I run outside of the airport. I have a tradition whenever I am on a 4-hour layover in Ft. Lauderdale. My husband and I run to this amazing restaurant called Gramps, just a couple of miles away from the airport where they know us by name, as well as Jaxons, where ice cream comes in portions as large as a football. We arrive a little sweaty, order a tasty omelet or a stack of pancakes, and then run back. Other "destination" runs could include a nearby beach or mall or monument of some kind. Or you can just go run and explore.

The only tricky part is finding a pathway or route that safely takes you from the airport exit (at baggage claim) to where you want to go. Not every airport is like LAX, which has sidewalks leading right out of the airport to long stretches of excellent running real estate. But in almost every place I have tried it, from Frankfurt to Trinidad and Tobago, finding that running route is not that hard.

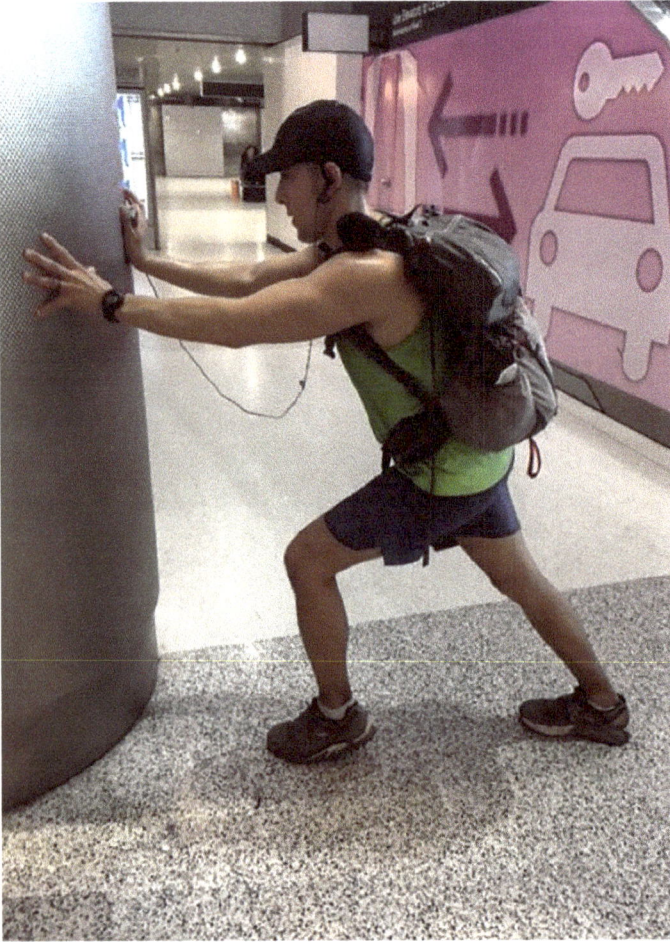

Baggage Storage

So, what about your stuff? If you didn't quite pack as efficiently as you meant to or simply have too much gear to run with, check out the baggage storage facilities in most airports, as I mentioned earlier. The airport storage in the Barcelona airport, for example, will run you about 10 Euros for several hours of storage, last time I checked. In Miami, it's only \$9 for the entire day per bag (keep in mind these prices are subject to change—so do some research). This is a care-free and safe way to deposit your items, allowing you to run outside uninhibited or even inside if you really don't want to carry a backpack while you do your terminal-running. Just remember to keep with you some form of ID and a small amount of money (for a taxi or water if needed), especially if you are going for a run in a foreign country.

Other Running Tips

Always study a bit about the security of the area where you plan to run, and if your run happens in the middle of the daylight hours, use some of that sunscreen and hat that you brought with you. I would avoid running outside at night unless you really know the area.

Also keep in mind that you may be arriving back to the airport a little (or a lot) sweaty. Not a problem. You can clean up before you pass through security; though if you plan to do more exercise once in the terminal, this may not make sense. If you do go through airport security in your sweaty running clothes, remember that the x-ray machine may detect the wetness on your clothes and flag it to the agent. Again, not a problem; this may mean you might require an extra pat down. Once in Ft. Lauderdale, I recall my pat down was quite "thorough." I almost asked the agent if he was planning to buy me dinner afterwards! Of course I didn't really ask; security should be taken seriously.

CHAPTER VI
Hygiene

THIS IS PERHAPS my favorite section to write, as I tend to get the most questions on how to manage cleanliness. One of my colleagues asked me the other day, "but sir, don't you get too sweaty and smelly?"

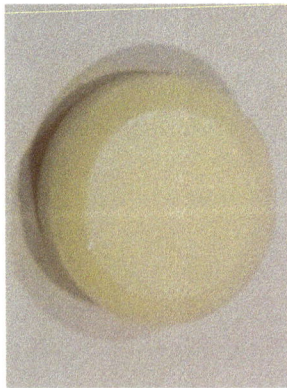

First of all, sure I do get sweaty. This is the hallmark of a really good workout vs. just doing some light calorie burning; nothing wrong with the latter though. Remember, it's all about goals. But the good news is there are many options here. First, some key items to always carry with you in your backpack:

- Small hand towel and/or baby wipes
- Small soap
- Small plastic grocery store bag
- Fresh shirt, socks, and underwear
- Small after-shave cream or cream (Gillette makes a 2.5-ounce after-shave that is only around $3).

---

*A **Stanford University study** found that older runners' knees were no less healthy than those of people who don't run.*

http://www.health.com

For me, I sweat profusely. I blame it on my Ecuadorian grandma who can't even vacuum her house without drenching a shirt. So, when I do my airport workouts, I really go hard. This means I drench a shirt, my running shorts, and often my socks. Luckily, since I packed sensibly and am already wearing my running shorts, I simply have to take off my pants, put on my headphones, and let the sweat roll. Then I have a change of clothes ready in my backpack for afterwards. All I need is a way to clean up.

Naturally, if you are a Platinum Star Alliance member, you might find yourself with access to premium lounges that have everything from buffet food options to showers to sleep quarters. But for most of us traveling on a budget (or on the U.S. Government's dime), these fancy lounges that can run as much as $50 or more per entry really aren't a viable option. In some cases, like the Frankfurt airport, you can pay 10-12 Euros to use a shower facility. And at the Dallas-Fort Worth airport, they have Minute Suites where you can pay to take a nap and/or shower for a short period of time. These aren't bad options, and I have found them to be relatively clean. But not all airports have such options.

http://minutesuites.com/locations/dfw-international-airport/

The next best place to clean up: the family restrooms which you can usually find near the male or female-only restrooms. These small rooms give you the privacy to clean up without your foot accidentally falling into the toilet or having to change your socks next to a guy who's unloading into his bathroom stall like the scene from Dumb and Dumber. Disabled or family bathroom stalls also offer larger areas (and often a sink) to take care of your business, which is another option if there isn't a disabled person waiting to use it of course.

Your brain depends on your stomach to signal that it's full, but that message takes 20 minutes to be delivered. So slow down during meals, and you'll be less likely to eat too much.

http://www.washingtonpost.com

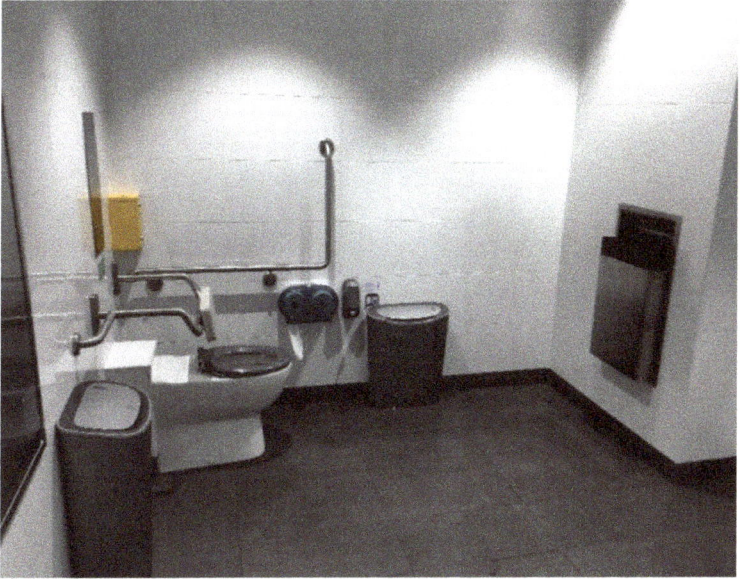

The first step, lay paper towels down so you can put your bags ON them, thereby keeping your bags relatively clean. Airports are already dirty places—one big fomite filled with germs. Think of the movie Outbreak (the movie theater scene). So, take a few seconds to place your bags on something other than the dirty bathroom floor.

Utilizing the door hooks found in most stalls, hang up your backpack or your dirty shirt, and use the sink to go to town, cleaning all the key areas. I always bring a small wash cloth and a little hotel-size bar of soap. With these items, and paper towels if they are available, I do the necessary cleaning. You can get fancy and remove all clothes and really go nuts, but just make sure to place paper towels around the sink to avoid making a mess for the cleaning staff.

I often stick a paper towel or two in the top and back of my shorts as I clean up, knowing the soapy water will travel south, and there's no need to make my wet clothes any wetter. And I often remove my shoes for the same reasons (always stepping on paper towels to avoid touching the floor). Apply some of that travel-size deodorant, though you may want to wait to do this last so your body has time to cool down first. You can fix your hair and put on some of that face cream you snagged from your last hotel-stay (flying dries out your skin!), and you are on your way.

Once clean, all you have to do is change into your second shirt (a fresh pair of underwear). In fact, you can change into anything you want. For those who like to fly in style, go ahead and change into those designer pants and Italian leather shoes if you really want to … or not. Your exercise regime need not affect the quality or style of clothing you choose to fly in—though some folks will find more comfortable and casual "flying" clothes to be more optimal.

Remember to put your sweaty clothes in the plastic bag; it will keep the rest of your items in the backpack protected. One tip: when you eventually get to that hotel or return home, don't forget to take those sweaty clothes out of the plastic bag to wash. The consequences of forgetting this for weeks on end … let's just say it doesn't end well.

Still worried about smells? Here are a few extra tips. As you stroll down the airport, refreshed and cooling down, don't hesitate to sample a cologne or perfume at one of the endless boutiques and duty free shops. One or two sample sprays, as you "consider" buying the item for the sake of shop clerks, and you might find yourself the best smelling passenger on the plane. Though remember if you put too much on, you might cause that middle school teacher seated next to you to start sneezing!

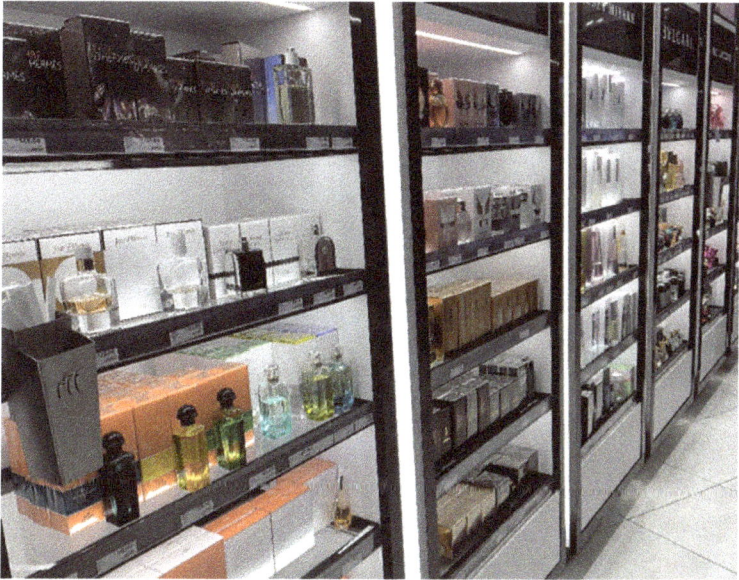

Oh and a few drops of baby powder that I put into my running shoes before I left to the airport ensure my feet don't stink up the plane. It's ironic how often I get compliments from other passengers about my good smells. Now, you might not be clean enough to go to a formal dinner with the Royal Family, but you will get the job done.

Lastly, if all you plan to do is a little light sweating, none of these "mini showers" will be necessary. You could, for example, use baby wipes to clean up the key areas like your neck, face, and even armpits. This is an excellent way to mop up some sweat, refresh your skin, and get you smelling clean again. Or you can simply put a few paper towels down your shirt to absorb the little bit of sweat. This will keep your shirt dry and from smelling. Getting worried that you will become a spectacle? Read the next section!!

CHAPTER VII
The Stares, the Shame!

REMEMBERING THE OLD adage from Mom, "they are just jealous" can explain a lot. In fact, this response appropriately describes the reaction you will see in many of your fellow passengers. As the man seated near you chows down on a Wendy's burger, glaring at you (oops, did he see that bit of ketchup fall onto his new Brooks Brothers shirt?), don't give his reaction a second thought. As the teenager girls giggle hysterically as your sweat falls from you onto the floor like a dripping faucet, don't "sweat" their ridicule.

Most of the time, other passengers will at worst feel resentment towards you because they know you are doing what they know they should be doing. Others may be turned off by seeing you kill those triceps dips on the airport chair (remember to bring a paper towel to wipe it off!).

But most people are just curious and interested, and in some cases, they will probably admire you for taking the initiative to do something healthy while so many others choose not to do so. I kid you not: I was once going to town with my resistance cords in the airport, sweat flying off of me, and

I just happened to look up to see Alex Trebek staring at me in a nearby seat, with a curious smile on his face. At least it looked like him!

The bottom line is that those who seriously exercise in airports CAN be a bit of a spectacle. Your short shorts, tank tops, and intense workout don't quite fit with what people expect in airport, even though if you really look around, you would find the most fascinating and strange sights in airports. Ever come across that woman in tights, clipping her toenails by Gate 24B? Remember that old dirty blanket on the floor of the airport you casually pass by on the way to bathroom? Oh wait, there's a human being sleeping there before his flight!

Doing something unique and unusual may be intimidating for some folks at first. As someone who has run shirtless in several Caribbean nations, I am often surprised by the reaction of some people who aren't used to seeing something out of the ordinary. My recommendation is that you try not to pay much attention. I just do my own thing and don't really worry about what others think about my exercise.

This is not to say that you should go out of your way to raise attention to yourself. There is no reason to not at least try to keep somewhat of a low profile, which may mean finding an emptier part of the terminal to do your exercises, facing the windows (and away from the crowded hallways), and being discreet whenever possible. As mentioned elsewhere in this book, it is important to follow rules and instructions from those in charge.

Ultimately, airports are a smorgasbord of strange and curious events, so in many ways, your 5K jog down the terminal isn't really that out of the ordinary at all. And if people notice, consider the fact that you might be inspiring them to get off their bums and do something more than just check that Facebook account for the 10th time in the last minute. Sorry, Dave, he just hasn't written you a text since you last checked. Don't pay attention to them, and it won't bother you. You might even feel some much-deserved pride.

CHAPTER VIII
Last Tips

DON'T FORGET TO hydrate. Flying already dehydrates the body, so don't make it worse by not drinking enough fluids. For the same reason, packing a travel-sized body lotion will help replenish needed nutrients to the skin after your workout. If you are really on a budget, there are many places in airports that will give free water. If you see a Chili's or Burger King or even Panda Express, ask for a small cup of water. Most times they will give it to you free of charge, even if you don't buy anything.

Bring your own food, unless you are flying First Class of course! This way, you get to save time and money at the airport, and you get to control the content of the food you eat.

Don't be hard on yourself if you can't commit to airport workouts every time. If you make some goals, put in the effort, and try, you will find you can make it work more often than not. Other times, it is nice to just relax.

Clean up after yourself. If you get sweat on the floor, wipe it up. Same goes for the airport seats. If you splash soapy water all of the sink mirror, wipe it down. You don't need to worry about making everything "Mr. Clean-clean." But it only takes a few seconds to wipe up your mess.

Just Try It (a Couple of Times)

Exercising in airports and during layovers sounds like a lot of work to some people. But after a few tries, you get into a routine, and it becomes easier and something you can actually

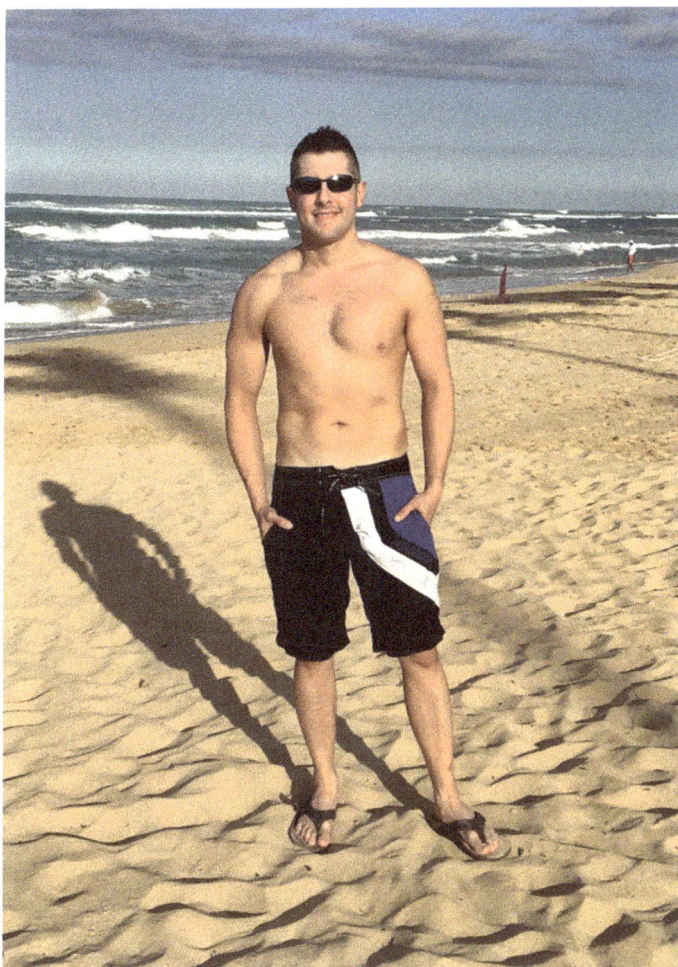

look forward to doing. Plus, a chronic lack of exercise can also be time consuming. Ask the guy overcoming obesity or the gal whose hemorrhoids won't seem to go away. Alright, so maybe you won't get hemorrhoids if you don't exercise in the airport every time, but you also won't be burning those calories, building muscle strength, and increasing your flexibility, which is healthy for your flying experience and in life overall. And once you start making healthy choices, even if others aren't, you might find it's easier to make those same choices in different parts of your life (like taking the stairs instead of elevators, biking to work, and running to dinner). After all, it's never out of season to have a beach body. Take it from a guy who lives in the Caribbean.

And understandably—storing four bags for a 45-minute layover or trying to go for a run with the kiddos may not always be possible, but there are opportunities to get at least some exercise in during your layovers. And if you are traveling alone, the options are plentiful.

So, the next time you fly, consider what you've read or learned in this book, and get going! It may change your life. And if not, hopefully you at least bought this book anyway.

THE END

(... or is it just the beginning?)

About the Author

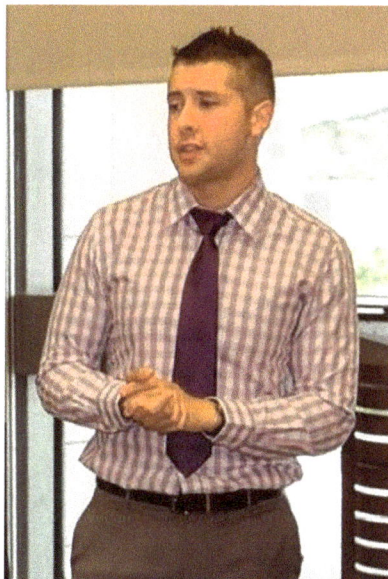

Originally from Nebraska and Colorado, among other places, Ken Seifert is a graduate of the University of Notre Dame and The George Washington University. He has traveled and served his country abroad as a United States diplomat and spent almost ten years living in Central and South America, Africa, and the Caribbean. An avid writer, Ken's previous publications include *The Rising Storm*, a novel published in 2007 and hundreds of letters to the editor and op-ed pieces have been published in such newspapers as *USA Today*, the *Washington Post*, the *Denver Post*, the *Miami Herald*, the *Austin American-Statesman*, the *Fort Worth Star-Telegram*, the *St. Louis Post-Dispatch*, the *Omaha World-Herald*, and the *Richmond Times-Dispatch*.

Ken is married and the proud father of two furry dogs. He spends his time traveling the world, exercising, or hiking in the beautiful mountains of Colorado. Otherwise, you will find Ken exercising in or around airports.

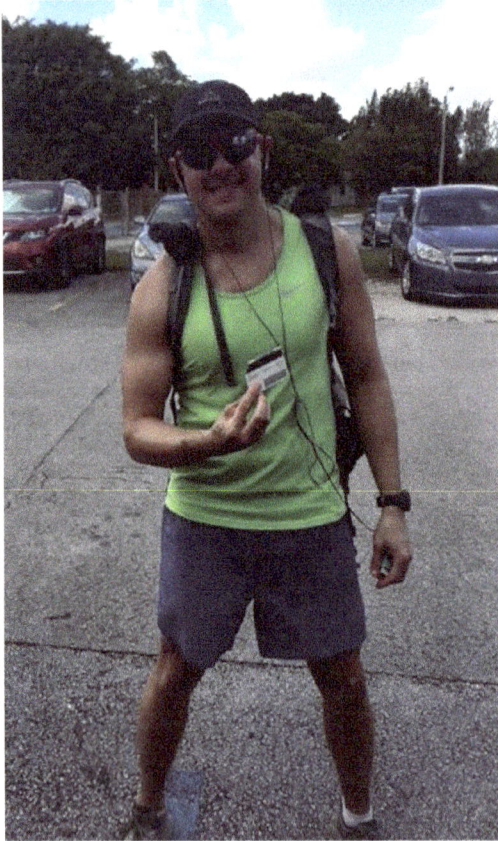

(Picture taken during one airport layover where author Ken Seifert ran 15 miles to the nearest DMV to get his license renewed. Anything is possible!)

Facebook friends needed! If you enjoy what you read, please "like" the official Facebook site for *The Complete Guide to Airport Exercise* at:

www.facebook.com/airportexercise

The author's self-esteem is tied to how many Facebook friends the website gets. Also, please write a review at your favorite on-line retailer. Thanks for reading!